THE *Skinny* PERSONAL
SPORTS BLENDER
RECIPE BOOK

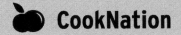 CookNation

THE SKINNY PERSONAL SPORTS BLENDER RECIPE BOOK
GREAT TASTING, NUTRITIOUS SMOOTHIES, JUICES & SHAKES. PERFECT FOR WORKOUTS, WEIGHT LOSS & FAT BURNING. BLEND & GO!

ISBN 978-1-911219-13-2

A CIP catalogue record of this book is available from the British Library

DISCLAIMER

This book is designed to provide information on smoothies and juices that can be made using personal blender appliances, results may differ if alternative devices are used.

Some recipes may contain nuts or traces of nuts. Those suffering from any allergies associated with nuts should avoid any recipes containing nuts or nut based oils.
This information is provided and sold with the knowledge that the publisher and author do not offer any legal or other professional advice. In the case of a need for any such expertise consult with the appropriate professional.
This book does not contain all information available on the subject, and other sources of recipes are available.
Every effort has been made to make this book as accurate as possible. However, there may be typographical and or content errors. Therefore, this book should serve only as a general guide and not as the ultimate source of subject information.
This book contains information that might be dated and is intended only to educate and entertain.
The author and publisher shall have no liability or responsibility to any person or entity regarding any loss or damage incurred, or alleged to have incurred, directly or indirectly, by the information contained in this book.

CONTENTS

UNDER 400 CALORIES   61

You may also enjoy.....

DELICIOUS, NUTRITIOUS & SUPER-FAST MEALS IN 15 MINUTES OR LESS. ALL UNDER 300, 400 & 500 CALORIES

ISBN 978-1-909855-42-7

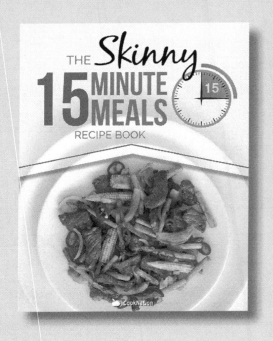

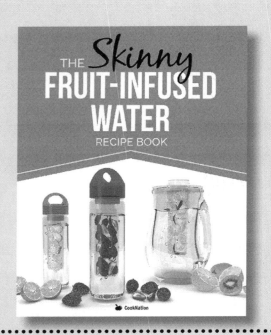

DELICIOUS, DETOXING, NO-CALORIE VITAMIN WATER TO HELP BOOST YOUR METABOLISM, LOSE WEIGHT & FEEL GREAT!

ISBN 978-1-910771-42-6

INTRODUCTION

Personal blending is the fastest way to create super healthy, delicious single serving smoothies, juices, breakfast drinks, protein & nutrition shakes.

Personal blending is the fastest way to create super-healthy, delicious single serving smoothies, juices, breakfast drinks, protein & nutrition shakes.

This no-fuss approach to a healthier way of living is a great way to increase your fruit intake, compliment your daily workouts, manage your diet or just have fun making great tasting drinks.

Blend & Go devices are hugely popular especially for the health conscious and those with a busy lifestyle. Using a personal blender couldn't be simpler…just add the ingredients as per our recipes, blend in the sports bottle then replace the blade with the leak proof lid and you're done! It's perfect for quick breakfast drinks on the go, gym nutrition or a meal-time filler if you are on a diet.

All the recipes in this book have been tested using the Breville Blend Active Personal Blender but they can be used for any of the personal blenders on the market.

Adopting personal blending into your daily routine has enormous health benefits. Balancing your diet with healthy nutritious drinks can help you lose weight as part of a calorie controlled diet, boost your immune system and help fight a number of ailments. Each of the recipes in this book are calorie counted making it easy for you to keep track of your calorific intake and help you achieve your 5-A-Day quota.

Using our recipes and your personal blender on a daily basis together with an overall healthy eating plan will help you feel brighter, rejuvenated, more focused and energetic. We hope you enjoy our recipes!

TIPS

Personal blenders are simple and easy to use. Follow these tips to get the most from your device:

- When using ice in your drink, always immerse the ice first in a little liquid. You can do this in the sports bottle with the liquid ingredients you are using such as a little water or fruit juice.

- When you are adding ingredients don't fill the sports bottle above the 600ml mark or max line.

- If some ingredients become stuck around the blade just detach the bottle from the base unit and give it a good shake to loosen the ingredients then blend again.

- Clean the blender base unit with a damp cloth. The blade, bottle and cap can all be placed in a dishwasher or alternatively wash with warm soapy water. For best results wash parts immediately after using.

- For stubborn ingredients that may have stuck to the blade or the inside of the bottle, half fill the bottle with warm water and a drop or two of detergent, fit the blade and attach to the base unit pulsing for 10 seconds or so.

- Use the freshest produce available. We recommend buying organic produce whenever you can if your budget allows. You can also freeze your fruit to preserve it.

- Wash your fruit and veg before blending to remove any traces of bacteria, pesticides and insects.

- Chop ingredients, especially harder produce, into small pieces to ensure smoother blending.

- Substitute where you need to. If you can't source a particular ingredient, try another instead. Experiment and enjoy!

ALL RECIPES ARE A GUIDE ONLY
All the recipes in this book are a guide only. You may need to alter quantities to suit your own appliances.

ABOUT COOKNATION
CookNation is the leading publisher of innovative and practical recipe books for the modern, health conscious cook.

CookNation titles bring together delicious, easy and practical recipes with their unique approach - easy and delicious, no-nonsense recipes - making cooking for diets and healthy eating fast, simple and fun.

With a range of #1 best-selling titles - from the innovative 'Skinny' calorie-counted series, to the 5:2 Diet Recipes collection - CookNation recipe books prove that 'Diet' can still mean 'Delicious'!

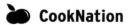 CookNation

THE *Skinny* PERSONAL
SPORTS BLENDER
Under 200 Calories

KALE SALAD JUICE

170 calories per serving

Ingredients

- 1 handful of kale
- 1 baby gem lettuce
- 1 apple
- 1 carrot
- Water

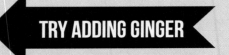

TRY ADDING GINGER

Method

1 Rinse all the ingredients well.

2 Remove any thick, hard stems from the kale and roughly chop.

3 Roughly chop the lettuce and discard the heart.

4 Peel, core and chop the apple.

5 Top, tail, peel and chop the carrot.

6 Add the vegetables & fruit to the bottle, making sure the ingredients do not go past the 600ml/20oz line or max line on your bottle.

7 Top up with water, again being careful not to exceed the MAX line.

8 Twist on the blade and blend until smooth.

CHEFS NOTE
Try adding a teaspoon of flax seeds for an extra boost.

LEMON BASIL JUICE

125 calories per serving

Ingredients

- 1 baby gem lettuce
- 1 apple
- 3 tbsp lemon juice

- 1 tbsp chopped fresh basil
- 250ml/1 cup coconut water
- Water

Method

1 Rinse all the ingredients well.

2 Roughly chop the lettuce, discard the 'heart'.

3 Peel, core and cube the apple.

4 Add the fruit, salad, coconut water & basil to the bottle, making sure the ingredients do not go past the 600ml/20oz line or max line on your bottle.

5 Top up with water if needed, again being careful not to exceed the MAX line.

6 Twist on the blade and blend until smooth.

CHEFS NOTE
Try using mint as an alternative to basil.

CARROT GEM JUICE

170 calories per serving

Ingredients

- 1 baby gem lettuce
- 1 apple
- 2 carrots
- Water

SWEET

Method

1 Rinse all the ingredients well.

2 Roughly chop the lettuce and discard the heart.

3 Peel, core and cube the apple.

4 Top, tail, peel and chop the carrots.

5 Add the vegetables & fruit to the bottle, making sure the ingredients do not go past the 600ml/20oz line or max line on your bottle.

6 Top up with water, again being careful not to exceed the MAX line.

7 Twist on the blade and blend until smooth.

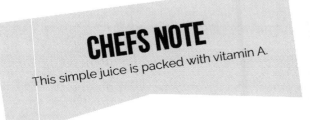

CHEFS NOTE

This simple juice is packed with vitamin A.

TURMERIC JUICE

135 calories per serving

Ingredients

- 1 handful of spinach
- 1 apple
- 1 carrot
- 1 tsp ground turmeric
- Water

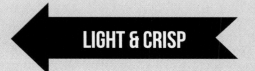

LIGHT & CRISP

Method

1 Rinse all the ingredients well.

2 Remove any thick, hard stems from the spinach and roughly chop.

3 Peel, core and chop the apple.

4 Top, tail, peel and chop the carrot.

5 Add the vegetables, fruit & turmeric to the bottle, making sure the ingredients do not go past the 600ml/20oz line or max line on your bottle.

6 Top up with water, again being careful not to exceed the MAX line.

7 Twist on the blade and blend until smooth.

CHEFS NOTE

Turmeric adds colour and spice to this unusual juice. Try a pinch of cayenne pepper too.

CHINESE GREEN JUICE

115 calories per serving

Ingredients

- 1 handful of spinach
- 1 handful of pak choi/bok choi
- 1 green apple
- Water

← ASIAN GREENS

Method

1 Rinse all the ingredients well.

2 Remove any thick, hard stems from the spinach & pak choi and roughly chop.

3 Peel, core and chop the apple.

4 Add the fruit & vegetables to the bottle, making sure the ingredients do not go past the 600ml/20oz line or max line on your bottle.

5 Top up with water, again being careful not to exceed the MAX line.

6 Twist on the blade and blend until smooth.

CHEFS NOTE

Pak choi is an Asian style cabbage which is now widely available in most stores.

GREEN GOODNESS JUICE

85
calories per
serving

········· *Ingredients* ·········

- 1 handful of spinach
- 1 handful of kale
- 1 pear
- 1 tbsp lemon juice
- Water

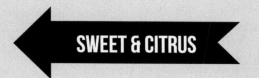

SWEET & CITRUS

········· *Method* ·········

1 Rinse all the ingredients well.

2 Remove any thick, hard stems from the spinach and kale & roughly chop.

3 Peel, core and chop the pear.

4 Add the fruit, vegetables & lemon juice to the bottle, making sure the ingredients do not go past the 600ml/20oz line or max line on your bottle.

5 Top up with water, again being careful not to exceed the MAX line.

6 Twist on the blade and blend until smooth.

CHEFS NOTE

Add a teaspoon of honey if you struggle with the taste of some of the kale based juices.

BRIGHT & BREEZY APPLE JUICE

115 calories per serving

Ingredients

- 2 handfuls of spinach
- 1 apple
- 1 tbsp lemon juice
- Water

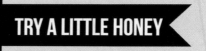

TRY A LITTLE HONEY

Method

1 Rinse all the ingredients well.

2 Remove any thick, hard stems from the spinach and roughly chop.

3 Peel, core and chop the apple.

4 Add the fruit, vegetables & lemon juice to the bottle, making sure the ingredients do not go past the 600ml/20oz line or max line on your bottle.

5 Top up with water, again being careful not to exceed the MAX line.

6 Twist on the blade and blend until smooth.

CHEFS NOTE

Give the bottle a good shake mid-way through blending if you find all the ingredients aren't coming together.

PAK CHOI JUICE

185 calories per serving

Ingredients

- 1 pak choi/bok choy
- 1 pear
- 1 apple
- ½ banana
- Water

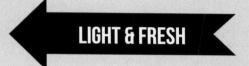

LIGHT & FRESH

Method

1 Rinse all the ingredients well.

2 Shred the pak choi, remove any hard bulb parts.

3 Peel, core & chop the pear & apple.

4 Peel the banana then break into small pieces.

5 Add the chopped fruit & vegetables to the bottle, making sure the ingredients do not go past the 600ml/20oz line or max line on your bottle.

6 Top up with water, again being careful not to exceed the MAX line.

7 Twist on the blade and blend until smooth.

CHEFS NOTE
Pak choi is a great juice alternative to spinach and kale.

CHIA ENERGY JUICE

180 calories per serving

Ingredients

- 1 handful of spinach
- 1 apple
- 2 tsp chia seeds
- 250ml/1 cup coconut water
- Water

LOW CHOLESTEROL

Method

1 Rinse all the ingredients well.

2 Remove any thick, hard stems from the spinach and roughly chop.

3 Peel, core & chop the apple.

4 Add the chopped fruit, vegetables, chia seeds & coconut water to the bottle, making sure the ingredients do not go past the 600ml/20oz line or max line on your bottle.

5 Top up with water if it needs it, again being careful not to exceed the MAX line.

6 Twist on the blade and blend until smooth.

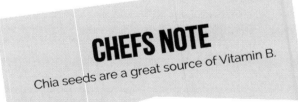

CHEFS NOTE

Chia seeds are a great source of Vitamin B.

APPLE & LIME JUICE

110 calories per serving

Ingredients

- 1 apple
- 1 cucumber
- 4 tsp lime juice
- Water

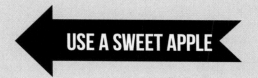

USE A SWEET APPLE

Method

1 Rinse all the ingredients well.

2 Peel, core & chop the apple.

3 Peel & chop the cucumber.

4 Add the chopped fruit, vegetables & lime juice to the bottle, making sure the ingredients do not go past the 600ml/20oz line or max line on your bottle.

5 Top up with water, again being careful not to exceed the MAX line.

6 Twist on the blade and blend until smooth.

CHEFS NOTE
Put some of the cucumber to one side if you can't fit it all in.

TOMATO GREEN JUICE

45 calories per serving

Ingredients

- 1 handful of spinach
- 2 celery stalks
- 1 vine ripened tomato
- ½ cucumber
- ½ tsp cayenne pepper (optional)
- Water

Method

1 Rinse all the ingredients well.

2 Remove any thick, hard stems from the spinach and roughly chop.

3 Chop the celery, discarding any tops.

4 Chop the tomato. Peel & chop the cucumber.

5 Add the chopped salad & cayenne pepper to the bottle, making sure the ingredients do not go past the 600ml/20oz line or max line on your bottle.

6 Top up with water, again being careful not to exceed the MAX line.

7 Twist on the blade and blend until smooth.

CHEFS NOTE

This is a really light juice, great for fresh summer mornings.

CITRUS SMOOTHIE

180 calories per serving

Ingredients

- 1 orange
- 1 banana
- 1 tbsp lemon juice
- Water

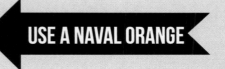

USE A NAVAL ORANGE

Method

1 Rinse all the ingredients well.

2 Peel and chop the orange, discard the rind.

3 Peel the banana and break into small pieces.

4 Add the fruit, vegetables & lemon juice to the bottle, making sure the ingredients do not go past the 600ml/20oz line or max line on your bottle.

5 Top up with water, again being careful not to exceed the MAX line.

6 Twist on the blade and blend until smooth.

CHEFS NOTE
Orange is the classic Vitamin C provider.

GINGER & PEAR JUICE

170 calories per serving

Ingredients

- 1 pear
- 1 apple
- 2 tsp grated fresh ginger root
- 2 tsp lemon juice
- Water

← ANTIOXIDANTS

Method

1 Rinse all the ingredients well.

2 Peel, core and chop the pear & apple.

3 Add the fruit, vegetables, ginger & lemon juice to the bottle, making sure the ingredients do not go past the 600ml/20oz line or max line on your bottle.

4 Top up with water, again being careful not to exceed the MAX line.

5 Twist on the blade and blend until smooth.

CHEFS NOTE
Adjust the freshly grated ginger to suit your own taste.

CUCUMBER GREEN JUICE

155 calories per serving

Ingredients

- 150g/5oz asparagus tips
- 1 apple
- ½ cucumber
- Water

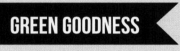

GREEN GOODNESS

Method

1 Rinse all the ingredients well.

2 Chop the asparagus tips.

3 Peel, core & chop the apple.

4 Peel & chop the cucumber.

5 Add the vegetables & fruit to the bottle, making sure the ingredients do not go past the 600ml/20oz line or max line on your bottle.

6 Top up with water, again being careful not to exceed the MAX line.

7 Twist on the blade and blend until smooth.

CHEFS NOTE
This is a really simple juice, add an extra chopped apple if you want a sweeter taste.

PURPLE JUICE

195 calories per serving

Ingredients

- 175g/6oz purple sprouting tenderstem broccoli/broccolini
- 1 apple
- 50g/2oz blueberries
- 1 carrot
- Water

Method

1 Rinse all the ingredients well.

2 Chop the broccoli.

3 Peel, core & chop the apple.

4 Top, tail, peel and chop the carrot.

5 Add the vegetables & fruit to the bottle, making sure the ingredients do not go past the 600ml/20oz line or max line on your bottle.

6 Top up with water, again being careful not to exceed the MAX line.

7 Twist on the blade and blend until smooth.

CHEFS NOTE

Purple sprouting broccoli is a great seasonal ingredient.

PINEAPPLE TABASCO JUICE

110
calories per serving

Ingredients

- 1 handful of spinach
- 200g/7oz pineapple chunks
- Few drops of Tabasco sauce
- Water

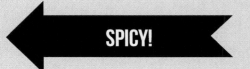

SPICY!

Method

1 Rinse all the ingredients well.

2 Remove any thick, hard stems from the spinach and roughly chop.

3 Add the vegetables, fruit & Tabasco sauce to the bottle, making sure the ingredients do not go past the 600ml/20oz line or max line on your bottle.

4 Top up with water, again being careful not to exceed the MAX line.

5 Twist on the blade and blend until smooth.

CHEFS NOTE
Use a little cayenne pepper or fresh chilli if you don't have Tabasco juice to hand.

FRUIT SLUSHIE

170 calories per serving

Ingredients

- 1 handful of spinach
- 1 apple
- 150g/5oz raspberries
- Handful of Ice
- Water

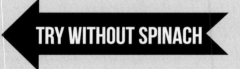

TRY WITHOUT SPINACH

Method

1 Rinse all the ingredients well.

2 Remove any thick, hard stems from the spinach and roughly chop.

3 Peel, core and chop the apple.

4 Add the vegetables & fruit to the bottle, making sure the ingredients do not go past the 600ml/20oz line or max line on your bottle.

5 Top up with water and a few ice cubes, again being careful not to exceed the MAX line.

6 Twist on the blade and blend until smooth.

CHEFS NOTE
Frozen cherries are also a good option for this juice.

TROPICAL BANANA JUICE

160 calories per serving

Ingredients

- 1 banana
- 2 kiwis
- ½ papaya fruit
- Water

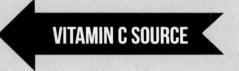

VITAMIN C SOURCE

Method

1 Rinse all the ingredients well.

2 Peel the banana and break into small pieces.

3 Peel & chop the kiwis.

4 Scoop out the papaya flesh, discarding the seeds and rind.

5 Add the fruit to the bottle, making sure the ingredients do not go past the 600ml/20oz line or max line on your bottle.

6 Top up with water, again being careful not to exceed the MAX line.

7 Twist on the blade and blend until smooth.

CHEFS NOTE

Native to tropical America, papayas are also known as paw-paws. They are sweet & juicy with a similar taste to peaches.

NUTTY BLUEBERRY SMOOTHIE

165
calories per serving

Ingredients

- 1 handful of spinach
- 1 carrot
- 200g/7oz blueberries
- 250ml/1 cup almond milk
- Water

← FIBRE RICH →

Method

1 Rinse all the ingredients well.

2 Remove any thick, hard stems from the spinach and roughly chop.

3 Top, tail, peel & chop the carrot.

4 Add the vegetables, fruit & almond milk to the bottle, making sure the ingredients do not go past the 600ml/20oz line or max line on your bottle.

5 Top up with water if needed, again being careful not to exceed the MAX line.

6 Twist on the blade and blend until smooth.

CHEFS NOTE
Strawberries are also good in this lovely smoothie blend.

STRAWBERRY CINNAMON JUICE

185 calories per serving

Ingredients

- 1 banana
- 100g/3½oz strawberries
- 50g/2oz raspberries
- 50g/2oz fresh pineapple
- ½ tsp ground cinnamon
- Water

Method

1 Rinse all the ingredients well.

2 Peel the banana and break into small pieces.

3 Add all the fruit & vegetables to the bottle, making sure the ingredients do not go past the 600ml/20oz line or max line on your bottle.

4 Add water, again being careful not to exceed the MAX line.

5 Twist on the blade and blend until smooth.

CHEFS NOTE
Fresh or tinned pineapple will work just as well. Use a little of the juice in place of water if you like.

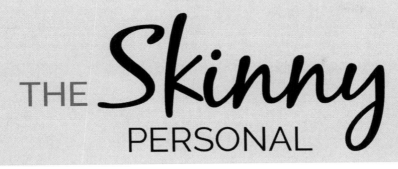

THE *Skinny* PERSONAL SPORTS BLENDER

Under 300 Calories

FRENCH BEAN BOOSTER

260 calories per serving

Ingredients

- 2 handfuls of spinach
- 50g/2oz French beans
- 1 banana
- 1 apple
- Water

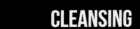 CLEANSING

Method

1 Rinse all the ingredients well.

2 Remove any thick, hard stems from the spinach and roughly chop.

3 Top & tail the French beans and roughly chop.

4 Peel the banana and break into small pieces.

5 Peel, core and cube the apple.

6 Add the fruit & vegetables to the bottle, making sure the ingredients do not go past the 600ml/20oz line or max line on your bottle.

7 Top up with water, again being careful not to exceed the MAX line.

8 Twist on the blade and blend until smooth.

CHEFS NOTE

This is great blast of green goodness. Adjust the quantities to suit your own taste.

SWEET NUT SMOOTHIE

275
calories per
serving

Ingredients

- 1 banana
- 25g/1oz walnuts, finely chopped
- 2 tsp maple syrup
- Water

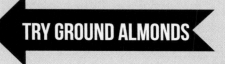

TRY GROUND ALMONDS

Method

1 Rinse all the ingredients well.

2 Peel the banana and break into small pieces. .

3 Add the banana, nuts & syrup to the bottle, making sure the ingredients do not go past the 600ml/20oz line or max line on your bottle.

4 Top up with water, again being careful not to exceed the MAX line.

5 Twist on the blade and blend until smooth.

CHEFS NOTE

For extra nuttiness try making this blend using almond milk instead of water as the base.

GOJI KIWI JUICE

295 calories per serving

Ingredients

- 1 kiwi fruit
- 150g/5oz fresh mango
- 1 tbsp goji berries
- 1 banana
- Water

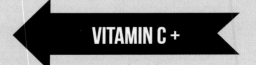

VITAMIN C +

Method

1 Rinse all the ingredients well.

2 Peel & dice the kiwi.

3 De-stone, peel and chop the mango.

4 Peel the banana and break into small pieces.

5 Add the fruit to the bottle, making sure the ingredients do not go past the 600ml/20oz line or max line on your bottle.

6 Top up with water, again being careful not to exceed the MAX line.

7 Twist on the blade and blend until smooth.

CHEFS NOTE
Try making this blend using soya milk instead of water as the base.

ROLLED OAT BREAKFAST SMOOTHIE

295
calories per serving

Ingredients

- 1 banana
- 1 apple
- 1 pear
- 2 tbsp rolled oats
- Water

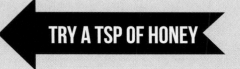

TRY A TSP OF HONEY

Method

1 Rinse all the ingredients well.

2 Peel the banana and break into small pieces.

3 Peel, core and cube the apple and pear.

4 Add the fruit, & oats to the bottle, making sure the ingredients do not go past the 600ml/20oz line or max line on your bottle.

5 Top up with water, again being careful not to exceed the MAX line.

6 Twist on the blade and blend until smooth.

CHEFS NOTE
This is a lovely cleansing blend, great at breakfast time.

35

ACAI BERRY WATER

295 calories per serving

Ingredients

- 1 banana
- 200g/7oz fresh pineapple
- 250ml/1 cup coconut water
- 1 tbsp acai berries
- Water

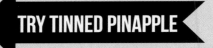

TRY TINNED PINAPPLE

Method

1 Rinse all the ingredients well.

2 Peel the banana and break into small pieces.

3 Add the fruit & coconut water to the bottle, making sure the ingredients do not go past the 600ml/20oz line or max line on your bottle.

4 Top up with water if needed, again being careful not to exceed the MAX line.

5 Twist on the blade and blend until smooth.

CHEFS NOTE
Tinned pineapple is also fine to use.

FRUIT CINNAMON COCONUT WATER

275 calories per serving

Ingredients

- 1 apple
- 1 banana
- 250ml/1 cup coconut water
- ½ tsp ground cinnamon
- Water

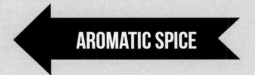

AROMATIC SPICE

Method

1 Rinse all the ingredients well.

2 Peel, core and dice the apple.

3 Peel the banana and break into small pieces.

4 Add the fruit & coconut water to the bottle, making sure the ingredients do not go past the 600ml/20oz line or max line on your bottle.

5 Top up with water if needed, again being careful not to exceed the MAX line.

6 Twist on the blade and blend until smooth.

CHEFS NOTE
Try adding tablespoon of coconut cream if you want a richer blend.

BERRY WALNUT SMOOTHIE

250 calories per serving

Ingredients

- 1 orange
- 200g/7oz mixed berries
- 250ml/1 cup soya milk

- 2 tsp honey
- 25g/1oz fresh walnuts
- Water

Method

1 Rinse all the ingredients well.

2 Peel the orange and roughly chop (discard any seeds).

3 Add the fruit, milk, honey & walnuts to the bottle, making sure the ingredients do not go past the 600ml/20oz line or max line on your bottle.

4 Top up with water if needed, again being careful not to exceed the MAX line.

5 Twist on the blade and blend until smooth.

CHEFS NOTE

Chop the walnuts before blending for a smooth finish.

MANGO CHARD SMOOTHIE

240 calories per serving

Ingredients

- 1 small handful Swiss chard leaves
- 1 banana
- 200g/7oz fresh mango chunks
- Water
- Handful of ice

FIBRE GOODNESS

Method

1 Rinse all the ingredients well.

2 Roughly chop the chard leaves.

3 Peel the banana and break into small pieces.

4 Chop the mango and add all the fruit & salad to the bottle, making sure the ingredients do not go past the 600ml/20oz line or max line on your bottle.

5 Top up with water & ice, again being careful not to exceed the MAX line.

6 Twist on the blade and blend until smooth.

CHEFS NOTE

Try using spinach if you find chard a little bitter.

PINEAPPLE BOOSTER

210 calories per serving

Ingredients

- 1 tsp lemon juice
- 1 banana
- 200g/7oz pineapple chunks
- 2 tsp grated fresh ginger root
- Water

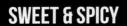

SWEET & SPICY

Method

1 Rinse all the ingredients well.

2 Peel the banana and break into small pieces.

3 Add the fruit and lemon juice to the bottle, making sure the ingredients do not go past the 600ml/20oz line or max line on your bottle.

4 Top up with water, again being careful not to exceed the MAX line.

5 Twist on the blade and blend until smooth.

CHEFS NOTE
Ginger has been used for centuries as a natural treatment for coughs and colds.

SWEET SQUASH SMOOTHIE

285 calories per serving

Ingredients

- 1 apple
- 200g/7oz butternut squash
- 250ml/1 cup almond milk
- 2 tsp runny honey
- Water

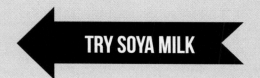
TRY SOYA MILK

Method

1 Rinse all the ingredients well.

2 Peel, core and chop the apple.

3 Peel, de-seed and chop the squash.

4 Add the vegetables, fruit & milk to the bottle, making sure the ingredients do not go past the 600ml/20oz line or max line on your bottle.

5 Top up with water if it needs it, again being careful not to exceed the MAX line.

6 Twist on the blade and blend until smooth.

CHEFS NOTE
Adjust the honey and almond milk to suit your own taste.

MANGO & PINK APPLE JUICE

280 calories per serving

Ingredients

- 1 Pink Lady apple
- 200g/7oz mango
- 1 kiwi
- Water

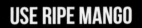

USE RIPE MANGO

Method

1 Rinse all the ingredients well.

2 Peel, core and chop the apple.

3 De-stone the mango and chop the flesh, discarding the rind.

4 Peel & chop the kiwi.

5 Add the fruit to the bottle, making sure the ingredients do not go past the 600ml/20oz line or max line on your bottle.

6 Top up with water, again being careful not to exceed the MAX line.

7 Twist on the blade and blend until smooth.

CHEFS NOTE
Pink Lady is a particularly sweet and tasty apple.

RASPBERRY MILK SMOOTHIE

299 calories per serving

Ingredients

- 1 banana
- 200g/7oz raspberries
- 250ml/1 cup semi skimmed milk
- Water

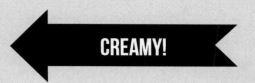

CREAMY!

Method

1 Rinse all the ingredients well.

2 Peel the banana and break into small pieces.

3 Add the fruit & milk to the bottle, making sure the ingredients do not go past the 600ml/20oz line or max line on your bottle.

4 Top up with water if needed, again being careful not to exceed the MAX line.

5 Twist on the blade and blend until smooth.

CHEFS NOTE
Add more banana for extra creaminess.

SPRING GREEN SMOOTHIE

230 calories per serving

Ingredients

- 1 handful of spring greens
- 1 baby gem lettuce
- 1 banana
- 1 apple
- Water

LIGHT & FRESH

Method

1 Rinse all the ingredients well.

2 Remove any thick, hard stems from the spring greens and roughly chop.

3 Chop the lettuce, discard the heart.

4 Peel the banana and break into small pieces.

5 Peel, core and chop the apple.

6 Add the vegetables & fruit to the bottle, making sure the ingredients do not go past the 600ml/20oz line or max line on your bottle.

7 Top up with water, again being careful not to exceed the MAX line.

8 Twist on the blade and blend until smooth.

CHEFS NOTE
Fast and fresh this is a lovely light juice.

GOOD GREEN GRAPE JUICE

220 calories per serving

Ingredients

- 1 handful of spinach
- 1 apple
- 200g/7oz green seedless grapes
- Water

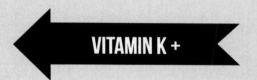

Method

1 Rinse all the ingredients well.

2 Remove any thick, hard stems from the spinach and roughly chop.

3 Peel, core and chop the apple.

4 Remove the stalks from the grapes.

5 Add the vegetables & fruit to the bottle, making sure the ingredients do not go past the 600ml/20oz line or max line on your bottle.

6 Top up with water, again being careful not to exceed the MAX line.

7 Twist on the blade and blend until smooth.

CHEFS NOTE
Red grapes are just as good in this juice.

GRAPEFRUIT SWEET JUICE

240 calories per serving

Ingredients

- 1 grapefruit
- 200g/7oz pineapple chunks
- 1 tbsp honey
- Water

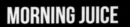 **MORNING JUICE**

Method

1 Rinse all the ingredients well.

2 Peel and chop the grapefruit, discarding any seeds.

3 Add the fruit & honey to the bottle, making sure the ingredients do not go past the 600ml/20oz line or max line on your bottle.

4 Top up with water, again being careful not to exceed the MAX line.

5 Twist on the blade and blend until smooth.

CHEFS NOTE

Pink grapefruit is a particularly good ingredient for juices.

APPLE CRANBERRY JUICE

295 calories per serving

Ingredients

- 2 apples
- 1 tbsp lemon juice
- 200g/7oz fresh cranberries
- Water

TRY FROZEN CRANBERRIES

Method

1 Rinse all the ingredients well.

2 Peel, core and chop the apples.

3 Add the fruit & lemon juice to the bottle, making sure the ingredients do not go past the 600ml/20oz line or max line on your bottle.

4 Top up with water, again being careful not to exceed the MAX line.

5 Twist on the blade and blend until smooth.

CHEFS NOTE

Adjust the quantity of lemon juice to suit your own taste.

CITRUS CARROT JUICE

210
calories per
serving

Ingredients

- 1 orange
- 1 apple
- 1 carrot
- 1 tbsp fresh chopped flat leaf parsley
- Water

← ADD ORANGE ZEST

Method

1 Rinse all the ingredients well.

2 Peel the orange and chop, discard the seeds.

3 Peel, core and chop the apple.

4 Top, tail, peel & chop the carrot.

5 Add the vegetables, fruit & parsley to the bottle, making sure the ingredients do not go past the 600ml/20oz line or max line on your bottle.

6 Top up with water, again being careful not to exceed the MAX line.

7 Twist on the blade and blend until smooth.

CHEFS NOTE
Adjust the quantity of fresh parsley to suit your own taste.

SWEET COURGETTE JUICE

230 calories per serving

Ingredients

- 2 apples
- 1 medium courgette/zucchini
- ½ cucumber
- Water

← USE SWEET APPLES

Method

1 Rinse all the ingredients well.

2 Peel, core and chop the apples.

3 Peel the courgette and cucumber. Top & tail them both before chopping.

4 Add the vegetables & fruit to the bottle, making sure the ingredients do not go past the 600ml/20oz line or max line on your bottle.

5 Top up with water, again being careful not to exceed the MAX line.

6 Twist on the blade and blend until smooth.

CHEFS NOTE

This is a subtly tasting super-cleansing juice bursting with fresh goodness.

KALE COCONUT WATER

250 calories per serving

Ingredients

- 1 handful of kale
- 1 banana
- 200g/7oz pineapple chunks
- 250ml/1 cup coconut water
- Water

TROPICAL!

Method

1 Rinse all the ingredients well.

2 Remove any thick, hard stems from the kale and roughly chop.

3 Peel the banana and break into small pieces.

4 Add the fruit, vegetables & coconut water to the bottle, making sure the ingredients do not go past the 600ml/20oz line or max line on your bottle.

5 Top up with water if it needs it, again being careful not to exceed the MAX line.

6 Twist on the blade and blend until smooth.

CHEFS NOTE

Coconut water is a great juice ingredient with low levels of fat, carbohydrates, and calories.

BANANA & SWEET PEPPER JUICE

260 calories per serving

Ingredients

- 1 sweet yellow pepper
- 1 banana
- 200g/7oz pineapple chunks
- Water

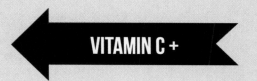

VITAMIN C +

Method

1 Rinse all the ingredients well.

2 De-seed and chop the pepper.

3 Peel the banana and break into small pieces.

4 Add the fruit & vegetables to the bottle, making sure the ingredients do not go past the 600ml/20oz line or max line on your bottle.

5 Top up with water, again being careful not to exceed the MAX line.

6 Twist on the blade and blend until smooth.

CHEFS NOTE

Use whichever peppers you have to hand but avoid green peppers as they tend to be a little bitter in juice blends.

DOUBLE APPLE HERB JUICE

210 calories per serving

Ingredients

- 1 handful of spinach
- 2 apples
- 1 tbsp chopped flat leaf parsley
- 1 tbsp chopped basil
- 1 tbsp lemon juice
- Water

Method

1 Rinse all the ingredients well.

2 Remove any thick, hard stems from the spinach and roughly chop.

3 Peel, core and chop the apples.

4 Add the fruit, vegetables, herbs & lemon juice to the bottle, making sure the ingredients do not go past the 600ml/20oz line or max line on your bottle.

5 Top up with water, again being careful not to exceed the MAX line.

6 Twist on the blade and blend until smooth.

CHEFS NOTE

Flat leaf parsley works better than the curly variety for this juice.

RASPBERRY & ALMOND JUICE

260 calories per serving

Ingredients

- 1 handful of spinach
- 1 banana
- 200g/7oz raspberries
- 1 tbsp ground almonds
- Water

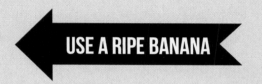

USE A RIPE BANANA

Method

1 Rinse all the ingredients well.

2 Remove any thick, hard stems from the spinach and roughly chop.

3 Peel the banana and break into small pieces.

4 Add the fruit, vegetables & ground almonds to the bottle, making sure the ingredients do not go past the 600ml/20oz line or max line on your bottle.

5 Top up with water, again being careful not to exceed the MAX line.

6 Twist on the blade and blend until smooth.

CHEFS NOTE

Try using almond milk in place of water as the base for this blend.

HERB GREEN DETOX JUICE

215
calories per serving

Ingredients

- 1 handful of spinach
- 2 tbsp chopped of fresh mint
- 2 tbsp chopped of fresh basil

- 2 tbsp chopped of fresh flat leaf parsley
- 2 apples
- Water

Method

1 Rinse all the ingredients well.

2 Remove any thick, hard stems from the spinach and roughly chop.

3 Peel, core and chop the apples.

4 Add the fruit, vegetables & herbs to the bottle, making sure the ingredients do not go past the 600ml/20oz line or max line on your bottle.

5 Top up with water, again being careful not to exceed the MAX line.

6 Twist on the blade and blend until smooth.

CHEFS NOTE
You can experiment with whichever mix of fresh herbs you prefer.

MANGO SLUSHIE

205 calories per serving

Ingredients

- 1 apple
- 200g/7oz mango chunks
- Handful of ice cubes
- Water

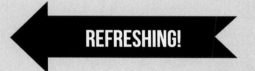

REFRESHING!

Method

1 Rinse all the ingredients well.

2 Peel, core and chop the apple.

3 Add the fruit to the bottle, making sure the ingredients do not go past the 600ml/20oz line or max line on your bottle.

4 Top up with the ice and water, again being careful not to exceed the MAX line.

5 Twist on the blade and blend until smooth.

CHEFS NOTE
Mango is a great source of vitamin C.

SPINACH MILK SMOOTHIE

290 calories per serving

Ingredients

- 1 handful spinach
- 1 banana
- 1 pear
- 1 cup/250ml semi skimmed milk

GOOD & GREEN

Method

1 Remove any thick, hard stems from the spinach and roughly chop.

2 Peel the banana and break into small pieces

3 Peel, core and chop the pear.

4 Add the fruit, vegetables & milk to the bottle, making sure the ingredients do not go past the 600ml/20oz line or max line on your bottle.

5 Twist on the blade and blend until smooth.

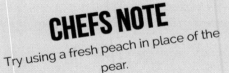

CHEFS NOTE

Try using a fresh peach in place of the pear.

TROPICAL ALMOND MILK SMOOTHIE

275 calories per serving

Ingredients

- 2 kiwis
- ½ banana
- 250ml/1 cup almond milk
- Water

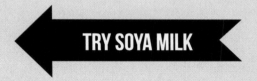

TRY SOYA MILK

Method

1 Peel and chop the kiwis.

2 Peel the banana and break into small pieces.

3 Add the fruit & milk to the bottle, making sure the ingredients do not go past the 600ml/20oz line or max line on your bottle.

4 Top up with water if it needs it, again being careful not to exceed the MAX line.

5 Twist on the blade and blend until smooth.

CHEFS NOTE

Use ripe kiwis to make the most of their natural sweetness.

CHERRY SOYA SMOOTHIE

265 calories per serving

Ingredients

- 200g/7oz fresh cherries
- 1 banana
- 250ml/1 cup soya milk
- Water

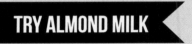

TRY ALMOND MILK

Method

1 Rinse all the ingredients well.

2 De-stone, de-stalk and chop the cherries.

3 Peel the banana and break into small pieces.

4 Add the fruit & milk to the bottle, making sure the ingredients do not go past the 600ml/20oz line or max line on your bottle.

5 Top up with water if it needs it, again being careful not to exceed the MAX line.

6 Twist on the blade and blend until smooth.

CHEFS NOTE

Fresh cherries are fabulous when they are in season but frozen cherries will work too if that's all you can get your hands on.

FIG & ALMOND SMOOTHIE

295 calories per serving

Ingredients

- 1 banana
- 3 dried figs
- 250ml/1 cup almond milk
- 3 tsp honey
- Water

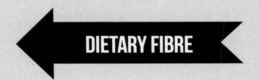

DIETARY FIBRE

Method

1 Peel the banana and break into small pieces.

2 Chop the figs.

3 Add the fruit, milk & honey to the bottle, making sure the ingredients do not go past the 600ml/20oz line or max line on your bottle.

4 Top up with water if it needs it, again being careful not to exceed the MAX line.

5 Twist on the blade and blend until smooth.

CHEFS NOTE
Soak the dried figs for half an hour in a little warm water before chopping.

HONEY RASPBERRY JUICE

220
calories per
serving

Ingredients

- 200g/7oz raspberries
- 1 banana
- 1 tsp honey
- Water

USE ANY MIXED BERRIES

Method

1 Rinse all the ingredients well.

2 Peel the banana and break into small pieces.

3 Add the fruit and honey to the bottle, making sure the ingredients do not go past the 600ml/20oz line or max line on your bottle.

4 Top up with water, again being careful not to exceed the MAX line.

5 Twist on the blade and blend until smooth.

CHEFS NOTE
Frozen raspberries are a handy ingredient for this simple smoothie.

THE *Skinny* PERSONAL SPORTS BLENDER

Under 400 Calories

CASHEW PEAR SMOOTHIE

SERVES 1

330 calories per serving

Ingredients

- 2 pears
- 1 banana
- 50g/2oz chopped cashew nuts
- Water

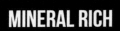

MINERAL RICH

Method

1 Rinse all the ingredients well.

2 Peel, core and cube the pears.

3 Peel the banana and break into small pieces.

4 Add the fruit & nuts to the bottle, making sure the ingredients do not go past the 600ml/20oz line or max line on your bottle.

5 Top up with water, again being careful not to exceed the MAX line.

6 Twist on the blade and blend until smooth.

CHEFS NOTE
Try topping up with semi skimmed or almond milk rather than water for a thicker blend.

BANANA & STRAWBERRY SMOOTHIE

315 calories per serving

Ingredients

- 1 banana
- 200g/7oz strawberries
- 250ml/1 cup soya milk
- Handful of ice

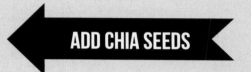

ADD CHIA SEEDS

Method

1 Rinse all the ingredients well.

2 Chop the strawberries and remove any green tops.

3 Peel the banana and break into small pieces.

4 Add the fruit & soya milk to the bottle, making sure the ingredients do not go past the 600ml/20oz line or max line on your bottle.

5 Add some ice, again being careful not to exceed the MAX line.

6 Twist on the blade and blend until smooth.

CHEFS NOTE
Almond milk works well in this smoothie too.

PEAR & AVOCADO ICE CRUSH

320 calories per serving

Ingredients

- ½ ripe avocado
- 1 pear
- 250ml/1 cup almond milk
- Large handful of ice

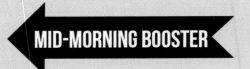

MID-MORNING BOOSTER

Method

1 Rinse all the ingredients well.

2 De-stone the avocado and scoop out the flesh, discard the rind.

3 Peel, core and cube the pear.

4 Add the fruit, avocado & almond milk to the bottle, making sure the ingredients do not go past the 600ml/20oz line or max line on your bottle.

5 Add some ice, again being careful not to exceed the MAX line.

6 Twist on the blade and blend until smooth.

CHEFS NOTE
Bursting with 'good' fats this smoothie will get you going in the morning.

SOYA & PINEAPPLE POWER

335 calories per serving

Ingredients

- 200g/7oz fresh pineapple chunks
- 250ml/1 cup soya milk
- 1 scoop protein powder
- Water

GREAT GYM BUDDY

Method

1 Rinse all the ingredients well.

2 Add the fruit, milk & protein powder to the bottle, making sure the ingredients do not go past the 600ml/20oz line or max line on your bottle.

3 Top up with water if needed, again being careful not to exceed the MAX line.

4 Twist on the blade and blend until smooth.

CHEFS NOTE

If you don't have protein powder use a handful of cashew nuts instead.

VITAMIN + JUICE

Ingredients

- ½ ripe avocado
- 1 apple
- 200g/7oz blueberries
- 2 tsp honey
- Water

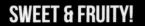 SWEET & FRUITY!

Method

1 Rinse all the ingredients well.

2 De-stone the avocado and scoop out the flesh, discard the rind.

3 Peel, core and chop the apple.

4 Add the fruit, avocado & honey to the bottle, making sure the ingredients do not go past the 600ml/20oz line or max line on your bottle.

5 Top up with water, again being careful not to exceed the MAX line.

6 Twist on the blade and blend until smooth.

CHEFS NOTE
You can use any type of sweet berry you prefer.

GOJI GOODNESS

340
calories per
serving

Ingredients

- 1 banana
- 200g/7oz mixed soft berries
- 1 tbsp goji berries
- 250ml/1 cup soya milk
- Water

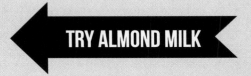

TRY ALMOND MILK

Method

1 Rinse all the ingredients well.

2 Peel the banana and break into small pieces.

3 Add the fruit & almond milk to the bottle, making sure the ingredients do not go past the 600ml/20oz line or max line on your bottle.

4 Top up with water if needed, again being careful not to exceed the MAX line.

5 Twist on the blade and blend until smooth.

CHEFS NOTE

Recent studies have indicated that goji berries may help protect against the influenza virus.

ALMOND PEACHES

370 calories per serving

Ingredients

- 1 banana
- 2 peaches
- 50g/2oz almonds, chopped
- 250ml/1 cup almond milk
- Water

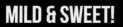 **MILD & SWEET!**

Method

1 Rinse all the ingredients well.

2 Peel the banana and break into small pieces.

3 Peel, de-stone and chop the peaches.

4 Add the fruit, nuts & almond milk to the bottle, making sure the ingredients do not go past the 600ml/20oz line or max line on your bottle.

5 Top up with water if it needs it, again being careful not to exceed the MAX line.

6 Twist on the blade and blend until smooth.

CHEFS NOTE
Tinned peaches will work just as well if you don't have time to peel fresh peaches

CEREAL HONEY SMOOTHIE

395
calories per
serving

Ingredients

- 2 bananas
- 1 tbsp rolled oats
- 1 tbsp honey
- 250ml/1 cup semi-skimmed milk
- Water

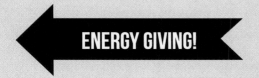

ENERGY GIVING!

Method

1 Rinse all the ingredients well.

2 Peel the bananas and break into small pieces.

3 Add the bananas, oats, honey & milk to the bottle, making sure the ingredients do not go past the 600ml/20oz line or max line on your bottle.

4 Top up with water if it needs it, again being careful not to exceed the MAX line.

5 Twist on the blade and blend until smooth.

CHEFS NOTE
You can add some chopped apple or pear to this smoothie too if you like.

CHIA BANANA BLASTER

365 calories per serving

Ingredients

- 2 bananas
- 2 tsp chia seeds
- 250ml/1 cup soya milk
- Water

OMEGA 3 +

Method

1 Rinse all the ingredients well.

2 Peel the bananas and break into small pieces.

3 Add the bananas, chia seeds & soya milk to the bottle, making sure the ingredients do not go past the 600ml/20oz line or max line on your bottle.

4 Top up with water if it needs it, again being careful not to exceed the MAX line.

5 Twist on the blade and blend until smooth.

CHEFS NOTE

Chia seeds are now widely available, they are packed with nutrients and are an excellent source of omega-3.

AVOCADO & SPINACH SMOOTHIE

370 calories per serving

Ingredients

- 1 handful of spinach
- ½ ripe avocado
- 1 pear
- 250ml/1 cup almond milk
- Water

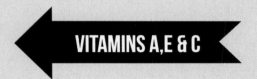

VITAMINS A,E & C

Method

1 Rinse all the ingredients well.

2 Remove any thick, hard stems from the spinach and roughly chop.

3 De-stone the avocado and scoop out the flesh, discard the rind.

4 Peel, core and chop the pear.

5 Add the fruit, vegetables & soya milk to the bottle, making sure the ingredients do not go past the 600ml/20oz line or max line on your bottle.

6 Top up with water if needed, again being careful not to exceed the MAX line.

7 Twist on the blade and blend until smooth.

CHEFS NOTE
Try substituting the spinach for kale if you want some 'hardcore' greens.

SMOOTH CITRUS BLAST

280
calories per serving

Ingredients

- ½ ripe avocado
- 1 apple
- 3 fresh mint leaves, chopped
- 1 tbsp lime juice
- Water

GOOD FATS

Method

1 Rinse all the ingredients well.

2 De-stone the avocado and scoop out the flesh, discard the rind.

3 Peel, core and chop the apple.

4 Add the fruit, mint & lime juice to the bottle, making sure the ingredients do not go past the 600ml/20oz line or max line on your bottle.

5 Top up with water, again being careful not to exceed the MAX line.

6 Twist on the blade and blend until smooth.

CHEFS NOTE
Creamy and light this blend is also good with a touch of spice. Try adding some freshly ground black pepper.

PEANUT BUTTER BLUEBERRY SMOOTHIE

385 calories per serving

Ingredients

- 200g/7oz blueberries
- 1 banana
- 1 tbsp smooth peanut butter
- 1 cup/250ml semi skimmed milk

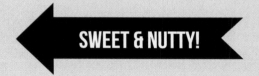

SWEET & NUTTY!

Method

1 Peel the banana and break into small pieces

2 Add the strawberries, banana, peanut butter & milk to the bottle, making sure the ingredients do not go past the 600ml/20oz line or max line on your bottle.

3 Twist on the blade and blend until smooth.

CHEFS NOTE
Soya milk or almond milk will also work well in this smoothie.

DOUBLE BANANA SOYA SMOOTHIE

370 calories per serving

Ingredients

- 2 bananas
- 2 tbsp low fat smooth peanut butter
- 1 cup/250ml soya milk

QUICK & EASY

Method

1 Peel the banana and break into small pieces.

2 Add the bananas, peanut butter & soya milk to the bottle, making sure the ingredients do not go past the 600ml/20oz line or max line on your bottle.

3 Twist on the blade and blend until smooth.

CHEFS NOTE

Use smooth peanut butter rather than the crunchy variety.

MANGO NUT MILK

355
calories per
serving

Ingredients

- 1 mango
- 1 banana
- 250ml/1 cup almond milk
- 1 tbsp ground almonds
- Water

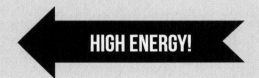

HIGH ENERGY!

Method

1 Peel, de-stone and chop the mango.

2 Peel the banana and break into small pieces.

3 Add the fruit, milk & ground almonds to the bottle, making sure the ingredients do not go past the 600ml/20oz line or max line on your bottle.

4 Top up with water if it needs it, again being careful not to exceed the MAX line.

5 Twist on the blade and blend until smooth.

CHEFS NOTE
You could easily use fresh chopped almonds in place of ground almonds.

TRIPLE FRUIT CINNAMON SMOOTHIE

390 calories per serving

Ingredients

- 1 peach
- 1 pear
- 1 banana
- 250ml/1 cup semi skimmed milk
- ½ tsp ground cinnamon
- Water

Method

1 Rinse all the ingredients well.

2 Peel, de-stone and chop the peach

3 Peel, core & chop the pear.

4 Peel the banana and break into small pieces.

5 Add the fruit, milk & cinnamon to the bottle, making sure the ingredients do not go past the 600ml/20oz line or max line on your bottle.

6 Top up with water if it needs it, again being careful not to exceed the MAX line.

7 Twist on the blade and blend until smooth.

CHEFS NOTE

Unsweetened tinned peaches will work just fine in place of fresh peaches.

CHOC-NUT POWER SMOOTHIE

395 calories per serving

Ingredients

- 1 banana
- 1 scoop protein powder
- 2 tbsp hazelnut chocolate spread
- 250ml/1 cup semi-skimmed milk

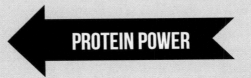

PROTEIN POWER

Method

1 Peel the banana and break into small pieces.

2 Add all the ingredients to the bottle, making sure the contents do not go past the 600ml/20oz line or max line on your bottle.

3 Twist on the blade and blend until smooth.

CHEFS NOTE
Nutella is a great hazelnut chocolate spread but any variety will work fine.

PEANUT PROTEIN POWER

395
calories per serving

Ingredients

- 1 banana
- 1 scoop protein powder
- 2 tbsplow fat peanut butter
- 250ml/1 cup almond milk
- Water

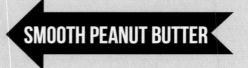

SMOOTH PEANUT BUTTER

Method

1 Peel the banana and break into small pieces.

2 Add all the ingredients to the bottle, making sure the contents do not go past the 600ml/20oz line or max line on your bottle.

3 Twist on the blade and blend until smooth.

CHEFS NOTE
Most protein powder comes with a measuring scoop. If not just use one level tablespoon of powder.

SWEET DOUBLE NUT SMOOTHIE

310 calories per serving

Ingredients

- 200g/7oz strawberries
- 1 banana
- 1 tbsp ground almonds
- 250ml/1 cup almond milk
- Water

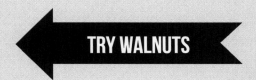

TRY WALNUTS

Method

1 Rinse all the ingredients well.

2 Peel the banana and break into small pieces.

3 Remove any green tops from the strawberries and chop.

4 Add the fruit, milk & ground almonds to the bottle, making sure the ingredients do not go past the 600ml/20oz line or max line on your bottle.

5 Top up with water if it needs it, again being careful not to exceed the MAX line.

6 Twist on the blade and blend until smooth.

CHEFS NOTE

In place of ground almonds try freshly chopped walnuts.

AVOCADO & BERRY ALMOND SMOOTHIE

375 calories per serving

Ingredients

- 200g/7oz raspberries
- 1 tsp honey
- ½ ripe avocado
- 250ml/1 cup almond milk
- Water

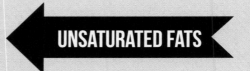
UNSATURATED FATS

Method

1 Rinse all the ingredients well.

2 De-stone the avocado and scoop out the flesh, remove the rind.

3 Add the fruit, avocado, honey & almond milk to the bottle, making sure the ingredients do not go past the 600ml/20oz line or max line on your bottle.

4 Top up with water if needed, again being careful not to exceed the MAX line.

5 Twist on the blade and blend until smooth.

CHEFS NOTE
Strawberries are also good in this smoothie.

CookNation

Other COOKNATION TITLES

If you enjoyed 'The Skinny Personal Sports Blender Recipe Book' you may also be interested in other '**Skinny**' titles in the CookNation series.

You can browse all titles at www.bellmackenzie.com

Thank you.

Printed in Great Britain
by Amazon